Blessed Is the Fruit of Thy Womb

Rosary Reflections on Miscarriage, Stillbirth, and Infant Loss

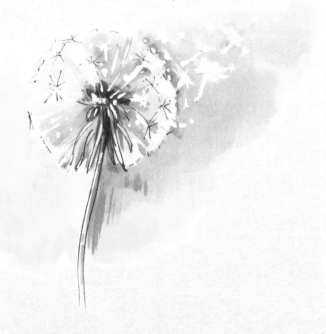

Dedication

This book is dedicated to all of the babies who inspired the reflections and the mothers who shared their children's stories with me. Your children live on in each of the men and women who use this book on their own healing journey.

Maria Christina	Louis Gerard	Marie Anna
Natalia Benedicta	Mallory Grace	Jackson
Cassidy	Carson Paul	Sarah
Carter	Patrick	PierGiorgio Matteo
Morgan		

...and my three miscarried babies, and Siena Therese, and Kenna LeeAnn.

Most precious little ones, pray for us!

ISBN: 978-1-68192-504-2 (Inventory No. T2393)
LCCN: 2019939981

Copy editing by Sibyl Niemann
Built by Steve Nagel

PRINTED IN THE UNITED STATES OF AMERICA

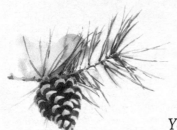

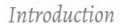

Introduction

You know you really shouldn't tell people so soon.
The rest of us get our hopes up and are disappointed when you lose them....

These words of a coworker stung when I shared the news of our second miscarriage. Did she really believe that it would be better if I kept this to myself and didn't bother my friends with our heartache? I wish that I could say that her attitude is unique, but the longer I travel the road of pregnancy and infant loss the more I realize that my experience is somewhat common. The only ones who truly understand its heart-wrenching nature are those who have endured it themselves. Yet they too are often unsure of what to say to another mom and how to offer comfort.

The good news, however, is that there is someone else who has a crystal-clear understanding of what it means to lose a child, someone who knew of the agony that her son would endure long before his eventual passing: the Blessed Mother, who stood at the foot of the cross and watched while her beloved son was scorned and humiliated, until he eventually died. Mary understands pregnancy and infant loss so deeply that she has been called the Mother of the Unborn. Mary desperately wants to offer us comfort and encouragement, and the mysteries of the rosary are her perfect tools for doing so.

The rosary is a straight line of communication and comfort for those willing to honestly experience the prayer and earnestly seek its blessings. In the months following the death of my daughter Siena, I unintentionally used the rosary as a reflection tool. As I cycled through the mysteries of the rosary each week, I began to see that there was a chronological journey of joy, sorrow, and glory that closely reflected the life of my own child. In Mary's joy and sorrow, I saw my own reflected.

Following our daughter's funeral, a family member had three rosaries created using funeral-arrangement flowers for the beads. It was perhaps six months after her death when those rosaries arrived on my doorstep. Now, as I continue to pray and heal, I draw closer to Mary but I also feel closer to Siena. Although I travel farther through time away from her physical presence in my life, the love I have for her has grown in my heart and the rosary has become one of the many ways in which I keep her close to me.

Inside these pages is a combination of scripture readings and reflections, prayer intentions, and questions. One way to use this book is to simply pray the day's mysteries, pausing at the beginning of each decade to read the reflection. You can meditate on the reflection or the questions during the decade and/or offer your prayers for the suggested intentions. The writing space opposite each reflection offers a place for you to record your thoughts, prayers, or even to write a note to your little one.

An alternate way to work through the text is to use it as a mini-retreat. Choose a notebook to keep track of your thoughts and reflections, focusing on just one mystery each day. Journal any thoughts the reflections bring to mind and reflect on the questions. In this approach, it would be best to start with the Joyful Mysteries and work your way through to the Glorious.

This book represents a journey of healing and a journey of love. It is a journey that I continue to travel myself. Throughout, I share many personal insights and experiences. You will also find inspiration from a diverse group of Catholic women who walked the road of pregnancy and infant loss. They share some of the ways the rosary was or became a part of their grief journey. While no two loss stories are the same, I want you to be assured that other women have walked this road before you. They too have struggled with their hope and their faith. They had days when they felt that this was simply too much to bear, and they could not imagine a day or a time when they would feel joy again.

No matter how much time has passed since the death of your child, be assured that Mary is waiting to welcome you into a deeper relationship with herself, her son, and your child.

The Author's Story

My husband and I were married on a sunny June day in 2002. We were excited to learn we were expecting our first child soon after our August honeymoon trip to the Black Hills, South Dakota. I excitedly scheduled an appointment with a local midwife and bought myself one of those pregnancy week-by-week books. Our excitement was short-lived, however, when I began spotting at eight weeks, the day before our first appointment. When our midwife confirmed that the baby had died and told me what to expect, she cried with me. Not knowing what to do, my husband and I drove to my parents' home three hours away. We shared the happy and the sad news together.

I passed our first child, visible and perfectly formed, in the basement bathroom of my parents' home, while my husband and one of our good friends distracted themselves with a playoff baseball game.

Three years later, after two uncomplicated pregnancies and deliveries, resulting in two rambunctious little boys, we had news of our fourth pregnancy. This pregnancy was different from the beginning. Our new midwife was following my hormone levels closely, but they never rose correctly. I delivered our baby in what could only be described as a heavy period after less than six weeks. If I hadn't known I was pregnant, I never would have suspected.

I remember being shocked by the intensity of my emotions. I had evidently convinced myself that our first loss was just a fluke and that I had done my share of that. Experiencing multiple losses was something that happened to other people, not people who had these two perfect boys, people who were young, healthy, and active.

During this time, our second son was having some health problems and was hospitalized more than once that winter for asthma-related complications. We spent two different weekends in February and every Friday that March inpatient or in the emergency room. Late in March, I woke up abruptly realizing that I had not had a period after my miscarriage. While we were "practicing NFP," I had never seen the wisdom in keeping charts if we weren't trying to avoid pregnancy, so I had no reliable record of when I could have conceived and therefore was sure that I hadn't!

Eventually, I took a pregnancy test and learned that indeed I was expecting again. Of all the things I remember about this time, the laughter at the news strikes me the most! Things progressed normally and in July we learned we would be welcoming the first girl into our family.

Then in August, after a period of no movement, we went in to learn that our daughter had died in utero at twenty-nine weeks. I was induced on August 28, 2007, and Kenna LeeAnn was born the morning of August 29 at thirty weeks. The months and years immediately following her death were, without a doubt, the darkest in my life.

If our first miscarriage was the catalyst for whole-heartedly embracing an open-to-life attitude towards children in our marriage, Kenna was our push towards the Catholic faith and for living our pro-life beliefs openly and unapologetically. We are converts who began practicing NFP a full five years before we even looked at the Catholic Church. To this day, I believe Kenna prayed us into the Church.

While she was working on that, God was busy blessing us with three not-entirely uneventful pregnancies resulting in three beautiful babies: another daughter in 2008, a third son in 2010, and a third daughter in 2012. When she was a baby, our older children would tease this daughter, Lucia Marie, that she was ahead of all of us because she was the first cradle Catholic in the family.

Lucie's pregnancy was very emotionally draining for me. I had never had three successful pregnancies in a row, and I spent many of the later weeks and months of her life waiting for the proverbial other shoe to drop. Then, on the feast of the Assumption, God gave me a conversion of heart that granted me the grace to keep going during the final weeks of pregnancy. This was my first notable experience with the

Blessed Mother and her incredible interventions, and my devotion to the rosary as a healing prayer grew from that day.

In 2014, my husband and I prayed fervently about continuing to grow our family. We had five beautiful children, and my later pregnancies had become more complicated. After returning very early despite ecological breastfeeding, my cycles were erratic and inexplicably infertile. Both of our living girls had been born via cesarean section and we didn't know how that would play into future births. It had never been our intention to be "done," but we were both worried that might be the case.

On Valentine's Day we learned we were expecting, and we kept our little secret together. Things were going along well and we chanced to tell just a few people around the eight-to-ten week mark. While visiting my parents, I began bleeding and my husband took me to the emergency room. After a quiet ultrasound, I sat in an absolutely silent room and watching the clock tick by while counting decades of the rosary on my fingers. I have no idea how many I prayed, but in the long wait for the doctor to return with the news I know it was a lot.

At eleven weeks, on April Fool's Day, I had my third miscarriage. Despite being much further along, I was fortunately able to still miscarry naturally, although it was a much more painful and involved affair than my earlier losses. My doctor told me later that I had what is known as a missed miscarriage, where I had actually miscarried much earlier in the pregnancy but for whatever reason had not begun the process of delivery until weeks later.

The next four months were filled with frustration with my body, which refused to return to normal: random bleeding patterns, crazy charts, no clear ovulation, but a slew of completely normal lab work. We eventually learned that I was expecting again, but it turned out I was much further along than anyone thought I should be, as I had negative tests and cycles in the meantime. To this day I'm not entirely sure when our fourth daughter Siena was conceived, even scouring over the charts later with a NaPro trained provider.

At approximately eighteen weeks pregnant, I had a serious bleeding episode and we made a middle-of-the-night trip to the emergency room with all five kids in tow. At this time we learned that our daughter was without amniotic fluid, and it was assumed that she would pass in the next few days either due to lack of fluid or preterm labor that could not be stopped.

God had another story to tell for her, however, and despite no amniotic fluid and a huge amount of medical uncertainty, she survived peacefully in my womb for the next nineteen weeks. Those months were a time of leaning on friends and family, much prayer, and the grace of the sacraments. In January 2015, Siena Therese was born into the arms of skilled neonatologists prepared to deal with the complications of developing without amniotic fluid.

They did everything they could, but in the end her tiny lungs had not developed enough for this world. Knowing this possibility, we had a priest on hand for baptism and confirmation, and she died peacefully in my arms after an hour and forty-five minutes. She was surrounded by the love of friends and family. We were all supported by a medical staff that was entirely respectful of our wishes for her. If death can be beautiful, Siena's was.

Grief was what grief was. It had been a very long year for all of us. More than a year had passed since we had prayed so fervently to add another child to our family, and that time had shown us a lot of heartache. I honestly didn't know if I was emotionally prepared ever to face another pregnancy. We prayed about waiting. We prayed about adoption. We decided at the beginning of Lent that we would pray separately about this intention for the duration of Lent and then return together to pray and make a decision as to what we would pursue.

After only a week or so of praying separately for guidance, my husband and I sat in bed one night and discussed that we had both been praying for another path but both had the strong conviction placed in our hearts that God was not done with our biological family yet. At my six-week postpartum visit, I asked my doctor what his thoughts were on the matter. He stated plainly as day that despite my having had ten pregnancies, three miscarriages, one stillbirth, an infant death, and three cesarean sections, he saw absolutely no physical reason that I could not have another baby in the future. More than that, he saw no reason to wait if we didn't want to and assured us that he would support us through any future pregnancies.

I think this was just what we needed to hear to feel open to that path. It wasn't that we weren't open to life—quite the opposite, in fact—but we were very hesitant about the potential health risks to me and future pregnancies (in the possibility of repeating any of the previous trials). If we had a serious reason to avoid, we genuinely wanted to know about it. In hindsight, I count this as one of the beauties of practicing NFP. Because of our faith, we had to talk about this immediately after Siena's death instead of putting it off. It wasn't an easy conversation, but it was a necessary one.

As a result of the conversations with each other and our doctor, our youngest son Tomas was born in late 2015. Because he was a few weeks premature and my fourth C-section, we spent a little time in the NICU, but his gentle spirit has brought an abundance of joy to our family.

For all too many families such as ours, being open to life also means being open to loss. While it is tempting to try to wrap each of our stories into a neat little package with a happy ending, the reality is that grief and loss are messy. Faith is often messy, too! As our children and our losses have grown and changed, we too have grown and changed. Our faith has grown and changed.

Each family who faces a loss will do so in their own unique way, and each will make different choices about how to integrate their child's life into their own. For our family, our Catholic faith has helped us find purpose in our suffering, celebrate the unique contribution of each of our children, and draw closer to one another. Our story is not about the so-called "right" way to handle miscarriage, stillbirth, and infant loss. However, Mary helped us find our way. My prayer for you is that with Mary's help, you will find your own way to carry this cross and to find hope in the journey.

If you would like more detailed information on any of the stories, they are each shared on my personal blog, www.workandplaydaybyday.com, along with many honest and raw posts about our grief journey.

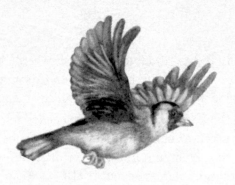

My Maria probably never would have existed if it had not been
for my meditating on the Annunciation, which led us
to take a leap of faith and God's creation of our precious daughter.
The night she was miscarried, my husband
and I stayed up praying the rosary as I labored.
The Baptism of the Lord was particularly meaningful as we prayed
and desired baptism for our child. When we finished our rosary,
our daughter was born, and we performed a conditional
baptism for her. She had probably passed away quite some
time before that moment, but knowing how much we desired baptism
for her serves to increase our hope to meet her in heaven.

—Jeana in Utah

The Joy of New Life

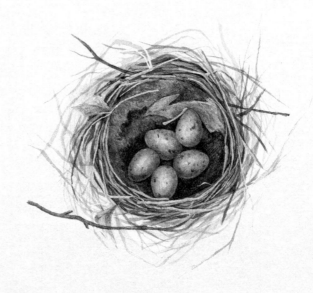

Annunciation

And Mary said, "Behold, I am the handmaid of the Lord;
let it be to me according to your word."

Luke 1: 38

When visited by the angel Gabriel, the scripture tells us, at first Mary was afraid (Luke 1: 30). Joseph too was later troubled by this news and concerned for Mary's reputation (Matthew 1: 18-22). John the Baptist, on the other hand, leaps in his mother's womb at Mary's arrival with the yet-to-be-born Jesus. Mary herself then rejoices in thanksgiving and praise (Luke 1: 46-55).

Many emotions can come with learning of a new pregnancy. My own reactions have ranged from joy and excitement to worry and anxiety, disbelief, and even fear. I have laughed and I have cried upon hearing this news.

When our children are taken from our lives too soon, it is easy to feel as though they were gone before we had the chance to make memories. While we may not have baby firsts and birthdays to share with other moms, learning of our child's life for the first time is a memory that is a part of his or her story.

The emotions you felt when you learned you were carrying a new life in your womb are an important part of your loss experience. Be it joy or sadness, make a note of what those emotions were. Consider writing them down. Where were you? Who was with you?

Offer this decade of the rosary for those who will learn they are pregnant today.

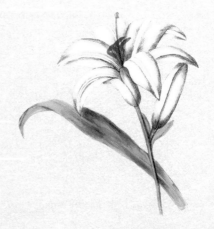

Visitation

And Mary remained with her about three months, and returned to her home.
LUKE 1: 56

Do you have a Mary in your life? *I do.* My friends Leigh and Jamie have again and again put their own lives aside to care for me and my family. It doesn't seem to matter if I angrily slam doors in their faces or call at 4 o'clock in the morning, or if they have needs of their own to take care of. They have visited me in the hospital, invited my children into their homes, and cared for us as no one else could. They have cooked countless meals and handed me twenty dollars for gas when I wasn't sure how I was going to get to the next appointment as medical bills piled up. Although they have different gifts, these two women have represented Mary for me on countless occasions.

I find it is usually easier to be Mary than Elizabeth. It is a challenge for me to accept both the love and charity of another person, particularly another mom with children. Imagine, however, that in accepting the friendship of Mary, Elizabeth was also welcoming Jesus into her home. When someone willingly puts her own needs aside to care for you, she too is bringing Jesus right to your front door.

Who was your Mary? Did someone put aside her own life and/or needs to come and care for you? What was that experience like for you?

Perhaps no one attended to your needs. How has that affected your relationships? Have you been able to extend forgiveness to those who have sought it? To those who have not?

Offer this decade for our culture's care of mothers: that we may be renewed in responding with an active, loving joy at the news of new life.

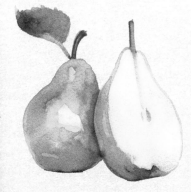

Nativity

She gave birth to her first-born son and wrapped him in swaddling cloths, and laid him in a manger, because there was no place for them in the inn.

LUKE 2: 7

No matter how far along you were at the time of your loss, your child had a birthday. Have you ever considered that? Your child had a birthday, just like Jesus did. Of course, that birthday probably wasn't what you hoped, planned, and dreamed of. This can turn birthdays into days of bittersweet memories instead of occasions of joy.

In addition to birthdays, there may be other special days, such as your child's due date, during which you grieve your child more strongly. While other families shop for presents and flowers, you stand painfully by and watch. Think about which days are the most difficult for you. Write them on your calendar and treat yourself extra gently on those days. Give yourself permission to buy flowers or treat yourself to a special "birthday" treat for your child. We always have donuts from a local bakery on our kids' birthdays, and we do the same for our girls who died!

Think about your family's birthday traditions. Are there any that could be adapted to celebrate the life of your child? Consider whether you would like to include others (spouse, other children, extended family, friends) in your celebrations, and how.

Offer this decade of the rosary for all those who will give birth today, particularly those whose children have already passed away or those who are expected to pass away shortly after birth.

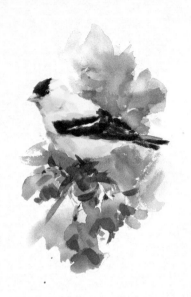

Presentation

"...and a sword will pierce through your own soul also,
that thoughts out of many hearts may be revealed."

LUKE 2: 35

Here in the middle of the Joyful Mysteries, we have our first glimpse at the sorrow that will follow for Mary and for Jesus. The prophecy of Simeon is one of the Seven Sorrows of the Blessed Virgin. A sword shall pierce her heart, just as it likely feels that a sword has pierced yours.

Simeon is a lot like the doctors who delivered bad news to us. I am struck by how quietly and gently Mary accepted her "diagnosis." She didn't yell at Simeon for sharing this bad news or hold it against him. She didn't go back to her hometown and tell her friends and family they should never go to this temple. I am forced to admit that I did not behave so admirably!

In my experience with our daughter Siena, I held her diagnosis against the entire health-care system that our doctors were a part of. It wasn't until much later, when my son was born and needed the care of the same NICU doctors that I began to realize how much holding that resentment against the hospital was harming my own healing process. In needing to trust them for my son's care, I found that my healing journey with Siena took a step forward as well.

Are there any relationships that need healing as you process your experience? Consider sending a letter of thanksgiving or of forgiveness. If you are unable to connect with that person directly for whatever reason, seek reconciliation through the graces of confession.

Offer this decade of the rosary for all of those who will receive difficult news about their pregnancy or child today and that all of those who will deliver that same news will do so with a spirit of compassion and respect for life.

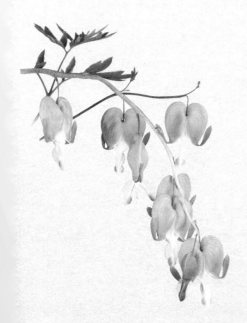

Finding of the Child Jesus

And he said to them, "How is it that you sought me?
Did you not know that I must be in my Father's house?"

LUKE 2: 49

For a few days, Mary and Joseph were missing Jesus. They literally could not find him even after searching high and low! It is no stretch for me to imagine what that must have been like for them as parents.

Imagine the extreme emotions that they must have endured. First Jesus was missing, but they were not even aware of his absence. Then how frantic they must have felt when they discovered him gone! Searching and seeking and not finding him. Finally, their joy and relief when, after searching, they discovered him in the temple.

In your time of grief, it is possible that it might feel like Jesus is missing. If you are struggling to find Jesus in your loss, go to his Father's house. Find a quiet adoration chapel, attend Mass, or go to confession. You may forget the words to the most simple of prayers, but just make time to sit with our Lord and let him come to you.

Give your relationship with Jesus a check-up. Is he missing and it's time to admit that you need to find him again? Are you searching for him but still waiting for him to be revealed? Have you reconnected with Jesus since your loss? How has your loss helped you "find" Jesus?

Offer this decade of the rosary for healing for those mothers, including yourself if needed, who have "lost" Jesus in the death of their child.

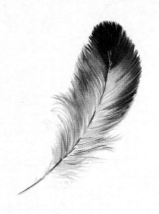

My daughter Mallory had a rare genetic disease and was born still. We prayed daily while I was pregnant and said the rosary. During the pregnancy, I was sad, but after she was born, I was angry. A LOT. At God, at everyone. A few months later, I started thinking about Mary. She lost a child too. The most perfect child. God, who was her Son. She had to follow him as he walked to his death on the Cross. She had to stand there for hours watching the life leave His Body. She had to bury a child. And live the rest of her life without him. Now granted, she was perfect. I was far from it. But in remembering that, it helped me. My Mother knew what I was going through. She had been there, and it was so much worse for her. I prayed to her for help in dealing with my anger and sadness. It brought a kind of peace. I was still sad. Now, almost nine years later, I still am. But I draw strength from my faith and from the example of Our Lady at the foot of the Cross and from saying Her perfect prayer, the Rosary.

—Amy in Kansas

The Light of a Child

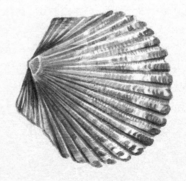

Baptism of Jesus

And behold, a voice from heaven, saying "This is my beloved Son, with whom I am well pleased."

After Jesus' baptism in the River Jordan by St. John the Baptist, the Holy Spirit descended upon him and a voice from heaven claimed Jesus as God's very own son. In baptism, we too are claimed as children of God.

But what of our child who has died? Baptism was something I struggled with greatly after the death of my oldest daughter Kenna, who died before she was born. At the suggestion of the hospital, but not understanding the spirituality or theology of the sacrament well enough, we asked for a baptism. It was explained (very gently) to us by our pastor that baptism wasn't something that could be applied to a person's soul after her body had passed away. We had a prayer and blessing of some sort instead, and it all seemed appropriate for the moment.

That being said, to this day, my stomach stirs uncomfortably anytime a baptism is celebrated, because I know that this is something that she did not receive. I have cried during or after Mass many times in the years that followed. Sometimes those tears fall privately later in the day, other times I am able to quietly slip out of the sanctuary and find a quite place, and yet other times I cry where I sit.

I am not entirely sure that I understand the teachings of the church on the matter of unbaptized infants and children.* However, I have also come to realize that it is okay if I don't understand and more than okay (in fact encouraged!) to lean on God's mercy and believe the best for her. I have come to believe that Kenna is in fact in heaven praying for us, and we have seen many instances of her intervention in our lives.

Baptism is only one of the many things that your child may have missed out on in this life. What are some of the things that are most difficult for you? How do you approach those struggles each day?

Pray this decade of the rosary for all of those children and adults who pass from this life without the graces of the sacrament of baptism. Pray for God's infinite mercy on their souls.

* Editor's note: A detailed study of this issue can be found in the International Theological Commission's 2007 document, *The Hope of Salvation for Infants Who Die Without Baptism*, available on the Vatican website. See page 61 for an excerpt.

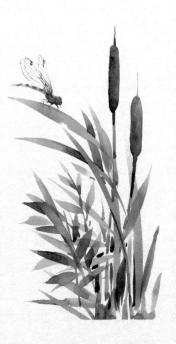

Wedding at Cana

This, the first of his signs, Jesus did at Cana in Galilee,
and manifested his glory; and his disciples believed in him.

JOHN 2: 11

If you have spent any time online following the death of your child, you have probably heard about many miracles: the miscarriage that never happened, the baby who came back to life after kangaroo care or hearing his mother's voice, the mother who carried to term after many losses. On one hand I am always thrilled to hear of these miracles because they result not only in the life of a precious child but in the conversion of many hearts.

At other times, however, it is painful and difficult not to understand why my family did not also receive such a miracle. Did we not pray hard enough? Did we not believe enough? Over time, I have come to realize that we too have been given miracles, just not the big one that I hoped and prayed for. Miracles come in many forms.

Our first losses were mostly mourned privately, but when our daughter Siena died her story was shared far and wide. For many months following her death, people shared stories with me about their own losses and healing. In being Siena's virtual voice and continuing to share her story, the miracle of her life continues to bring healing to others who are facing life after loss. In each of those stories of conversion, another piece of my heart heals as well.

What miracles are visible in your child's life? How can you share these miracles with others as a way to honor your child's life?

Pray for those in need of a miracle today. Ask that Mary help us all see God's great work even in our times of sorrow.

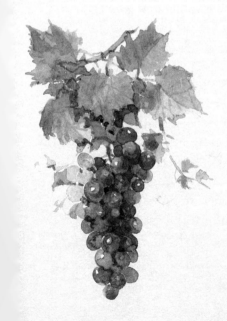

Proclamation of the Kingdom of God

But seek first his kingdom, and his righteousness, and all these things shall be yours as well.

MATTHEW 6:33

Jesus proclaimed the kingdom for all who would listen. It is now our job to do the same with our lives and with our words. That being said, it is a difficult task to proclaim loudly when something we don't understand has happened. Deep down we know the message of the Gospel is a message that is joyful. The path to heaven is open for us, and Jesus has shown the way! This makes us smile, but our child's death makes us weep!

Shortly after our daughter Siena died, we had the opportunity to participate in a filmed interview about our loss experience. Many people (including myself) who watched the video were surprised by the fact that I was smiling through most of the interview. I'm talking about our children who died—how could I still be smiling?

The truth is, I can't not laugh or smile, or at least make an effort to do so. Maybe this is a particular grace I was given or maybe just a skill that I have honed, but I don't know how not to look for the hope. And where there is hope there is a reason to smile and be joyful. Yes, two of our daughters have died. When I think of them, I absolutely think of this fact before any other and I am sad. To be sure, I have many hard days and know that I will continue to have hard days for the rest of my life.

Yet in Kenna's and Siena's lives were joyful moments as well, moments that we can laugh and smile about, regardless of the final outcome. In many ways, their final outcome is exactly why I continue to smile. In their short lives, they have achieved the kingdom of God, which is something I can only continue to hope, pray, and strive towards for myself and my living children.

Where can you find joy in your child's lifetime? Where is the hope? Consider how you can share this joy and hope as a way to proclaim the kingdom of God in your own life.

Pray this decade of the rosary for those who are struggling to proclaim the kingdom in their own life following the death of their child. Pray for them to find joy and to find hope.

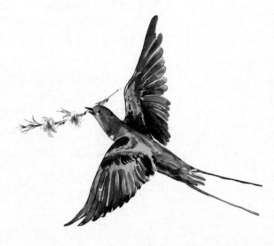

Transfiguration

And Peter said to Jesus, "Lord it is well that we are here; if you wish, I will make three booths here, one for you and one for Moses and one for Elijah.

MATTHEW 17: 4

The mountaintop sounds like such a peaceful place. When I read the full passage, I understand why Peter and James and John wanted to stay! Jesus knew, however, they had to come down from the mountaintop and continue the story.

Have you ever bargained with Jesus and asked him to just stop things where they are? Maybe you could just stay pregnant and then you wouldn't need to face your child's impending death? Maybe if you never leave the hospital, you will not need to face the reality that your child has truly died? Or maybe you could just stay home so that you don't have to face all the new babies at church?

The problem is, when we stay put we close ourselves off from our own transformation by the Holy Spirit. In order to continue the story, we have to keep living it no matter how unbearable that seems in this moment. That's the hard news. The good news is that just as Peter, James, and John brought Jesus with them from the mountaintop, so do we.

Peter, James, and John were all changed by their encounter with Jesus and the Holy Spirit on the mountaintop. How has your loss transfigured your own life? Are there things you have learned or could do to allow the Holy Spirit shine brightly through you?

Pray this decade of the rosary for the courage to leave the place you are and to go where Jesus asks you. Pray for the courage to be transformed.

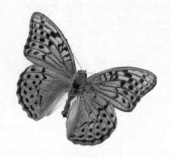

Institution of the Eucharist

Jesus said to them, "I am the bread of life; he who comes to me shall not hunger, and he who believes in me shall never thirst."

JOHN 6: 35

Like many Catholics, I love the Eucharist. Jesus loves me so much that he comes to me fully each time that I receive his body and blood. What an incredible gift he has given me!

My husband and I like to listen to audio talks from Catholic speakers and authors when we are taking long car rides. On one such trip, we slipped in "The 7 Secrets of the Eucharist" by Vinny Flynn. I can't remember all of the secrets, but when he began talking about how Jesus brings heaven with him, my husband and I exchanged one of those, "Is he saying what it sounds like he's saying?" looks. He goes on to speak about how those who have attained heaven are fully joined to Christ. They live in his presence full time. Not just when Jesus isn't busy living in the Tabernacle of our churches, but all the time. They cannot be separated from him and he cannot be separated from them. I knew that already, but I had never made the (entirely logical) step of wondering what happened at the moment of the consecration.

Jesus brings not just himself, but all of heaven, right to us. What does this mean? It means that when we celebrate the feast of the Mass as a family, we are truly celebrating with our entire family, everyone together, and Jesus is the one who makes it happen: a true feast of heaven and of earth.

The true presence of Christ in the Eucharist can be a challenging belief for many people but is also incredibly powerful once someone begins to make that step of faith. Meditate on how this understanding of heaven and earth's feast increases the miraculous nature of the sacrament.

Pray for those who struggle to believe that Christ is truly present in the Eucharistic feast of heaven and earth.

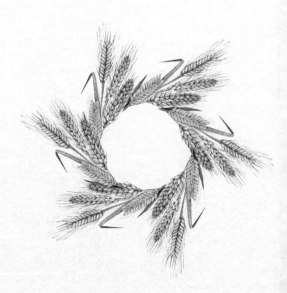

Carrying a child for weeks who was not expected to live was both the hardest and most beautiful thing I have ever done. The uncertainty of when and how Louie would be born and waiting for his birth were agonizing. For the first time, I could partially relate to how Our Lord must have felt during the Agony in the Garden. He knew his death was coming and He just prayed and waited. We knew Louie was expected to die, although we prayed for a miracle and the peace and strength to accept God's will. But unlike the apostles falling asleep and abandoning our Lord during his agony in the garden, we were not abandoned in our suffering. Our family and friends covered us in prayer and we were not alone. We prayed unceasingly for peace and we prayed the rosary every night as a family. We felt so close to Christ and so grace-filled during his birth and death, and we know it was because of the power of prayer. Carrying, loving, and holding Louie, our little saint, was the greatest privilege I have ever had and I wouldn't trade it for anything.

—Alison in Iowa

The Sorrow of Death

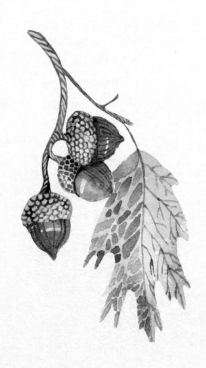

Agony in the Garden

And he took with him Peter and James and John,
and began to be greatly distressed and troubled.
And he said to them, "My soul is very sorrowful, even to death; remain here
and watch." And going a little farther,
he fell on the ground and prayed that, if it were possible,
the hour might pass from him.

MARK 14:33-35

Several things strike me about the passage above. First of all, Jesus in this time of suffering and sorrow did not surround himself with all of the apostles or the many others who had journeyed with him, but rather with only three. After the loss of a child, it is possible that you too may find yourself surrounded by only a small percentage of those who would have celebrated the same child's birth under more typical circumstances.

Even within his small band of trusted friends, however, Jesus still withdrew further. There were parts of his journey that he knew he must take alone, just as there are times when you will feel as though you must journey on alone. Jesus wanted his friends to keep watch with him, and his friends probably also wished they could do more, but they could not.

As Jesus wished the hour might pass from him, I know that you too wish that this was not a journey you had to be on. Jesus understands this desire and is, therefore, a most comforting companion. He will keep watch both with you and for you as you continue to grieve and to heal.

Sometimes we need to travel the journey of grief alone and other times we require the company of only a small group of others.

Consider where you are right now. Have you remained in the company of friends when you may have needed a retreat? Have you retreated for too long and now find yourself needing to reconnect with your support systems?

Consider who has come into the garden of your grief with you. Pray this decade of the rosary in thanksgiving for these people and the company that they provide you.

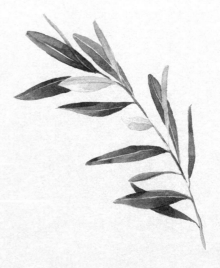

Scourging at the Pillar

Then Pilate took Jesus and scourged him.

John 19:1

I have to admit I was clueless when it came to what a miscarriage was. I had no idea that it was going to hurt. I didn't expect so much physical pain! Maybe if I had given birth before my first miscarriage I might have had an idea what to expect, but instead I was blown away. I sat on the toilet for hours—most of a day, in fact. Each time I imagined that the worst had passed and dared to leave the bathroom, I found myself rushing back.

The word *scourge* has two meanings. The first is to whip someone, and the second is to cause great suffering. Most people I have spoken with share my initial naiveté regarding the physical process of a miscarriage. It is a great suffering, the full purpose of which is to move closer to death. It is important to remember that the final chapter in Christ's story was not death, but rather life. By uniting our suffering (be it physical, emotional, or spiritual) to Christ's suffering on his journey to the cross, however, we can unite ourselves not only to his death but also to his resurrection.

What parts of your loss surprised you? Were you prepared for the physical pain and suffering that followed? How did you unite it to Christ's suffering? How can you continue to unite to it?

Pray for all those who are suffering physical afflictions.

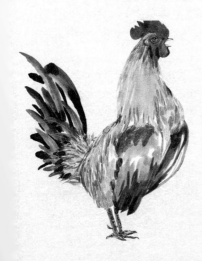

Crowning with Thorns

And when they had mocked him, they stripped him of the purple cloak, and put his own clothes on him.

MARK 15: 20

In most of the dramatic adaptations of the Stations of the Cross I have seen, Jesus is not only mocked but visibly humiliated at this scene. They have stripped our Lord of all of his earthly dignity, beaten him, stripped him, mocked him.

As a pregnant and childbearing woman we are often asked to bear a fair amount of indignity and immodesty for the sake of our children. Sometimes we even joke about various aspects with other moms. Yet the process of being literally stripped down to endure tests or procedures that we never imagined needing is no laughing matter. Some women are unable to miscarry naturally and need surgical assistance; others undergo extensive testing or surgeries for the sake of their unborn children.

In addition to suffering through procedures that may strip them of their own dignity, many women I've spoken with say their children were not shown the dignity of their tiny precious lives. When our children's lives are not shown dignity, it is much like being crowned with a crown of many thorns ourselves. No mother wishes to see her child mishandled, disrespected, or mocked.

It is easy to feel anger at the medical professionals who inflict these procedures upon us. Is there someone who stands out? Were there specific words or procedures you endured that could be improved? Consider advocating for yourself and future patients with a call or letter to the clinic.

Offer this decade of the rosary for the many medical professionals who work with pregnant women, deceased children, and medically fragile newborns, that they might provide care in a compassionate way that reduces physical humiliation.

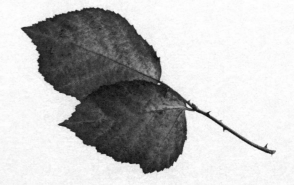

Carrying of the Cross

But Jesus turning to them said, "Daughters of Jerusalem, do not weep
for me, but weep for yourselves and for your children. For behold,
the days are coming when they will say, 'Blessed are the barren,
and the wombs that never bore, and the breasts that never nursed!' "

LUKE 23: 28-29

Can you imagine a time when a person would feel blessed that they were unable to conceive a child or carry him to term? Jesus says it will come, and others have said that in our current culture that time is already here. While many people seek to avoid the blessings of new life at all cost, there are others who quietly carry the crosses of infertility and repeat pregnancy loss. These are not light crosses.

Simon helped Jesus carry his cross. I can only imagine that Jesus was entirely grateful to Simon for his assistance, but how often in our own lives do we push away those who are only trying to offer a small amount of comfort during a trying time? Moms have human, earthly limits, and when we are backed against them, we have a tendency to push harder rather than yield to the assistance that we are granted.

I know I have been guilty of this many times, even complaining that the help offered wasn't what I thought I might need at that moment, or resenting the fact I needed help so much that I resented the person offering it!

You don't have to do it all alone. It's okay to let others carry you in their prayers and in their arms for awhile.

How have you responded when others offered you their help? Did you respond with humble gratitude or anger and resentment?

Pray for those who want to help like Simon but are unsure how to do so.

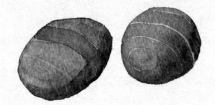

Crucifixion and Death

Then Jesus, crying with a loud voice, said, "Father, into your hands
I commit my spirit!" And having said this he breathed his last.

LUKE 23: 46

He breathed his last. Our daughter Siena breathed her last in my very arms with her father and me closely watching. We didn't know it would be her last breath, but we knew her time was drawing near. Mary too watched her son die. She stood by while Jesus surrendered all of his suffering in one final breath.

This is the point in the rosary when I always wish for Mary to pull me closer to her. No one can understand my pain of these losses better than the Blessed Mother herself. "Tell me how you survived this, Mary!" I cry out. It seems so entirely unlikely that a woman could quietly go on with her life, with her very ministry and calling, following such a tragic (and in her case public) loss. And yet that is exactly what Mary did.

Jesus surrendered to the Father and so must we. There have been so many days and times when I didn't want to get out of bed or to celebrate living with friends and family. The stubborn Finnish side of me wants to put my foot down and say, "Fine, I'll accept this, but I don't have to like it," to go on without really living. But to hold on to control is to skip the part about committing my spirit to the Lord.

Where are you holding onto control? What things do you still need to surrender?

Continuing to thrive after the death of your child can take many forms. You may be called to participate in new ministries, volunteer, or raise money in your child's memory. Maybe you will approach your marriage or other children in a different way.

Pray this decade of the rosary for guidance in your own "after" life.

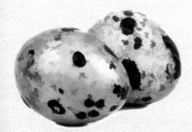

We are only human; who better to turn to for help

and support than the woman who gave her only son for us?

Peace comes in knowing She is mourning and holding you

while She joyously welcomes your child home.

—Sonia in Minnesota

The Glory of New Life in Christ

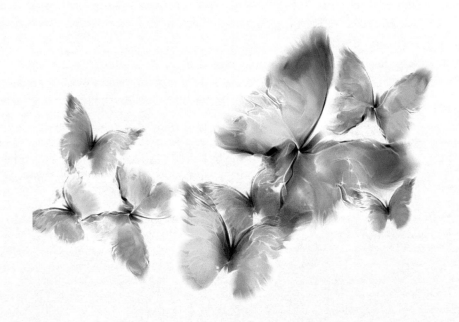

Resurrection

*And when they went out and fled from the tomb; for trembling
and astonishment had come upon them; and they said nothing to any one,
for they were afraid.*

MARK 16:8

In his death and resurrection, Jesus opened the gates of heaven so that we too may someday join him in the heavenly kingdom. This is a good thing, right? The disciples weren't so sure. They were afraid and astonished. Everything was different and they were overwhelmed.

Just because something good has happened, doesn't mean that we don't have to be afraid. We can have mixed emotions about our experience. Things are different for you now, just as they were different for the apostles following the resurrection.

Something ugly has happened in the death of your child. As we have been discussing throughout this text, there are also beautiful things in his or her life. As you continue to seek the blessings of your child's life you will likely face mixed feelings of your own. Life is going to be different now. Different can be a combination of things that are better or worse, but it can also just mean different.

How are things different for you now? What is better? What is worse? What is just different?

Pray for all those adjusting to different circumstances.

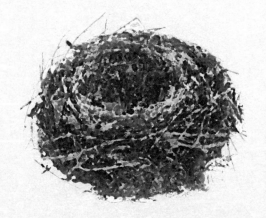

Ascension

While he blessed them, he parted from them, and was carried up into heaven.

Before Jesus ascended, he blessed the disciples. He blesses us too, although it can be particularly difficult to find those blessings during times like the loss of a child.

My first hope throughout this devotional is that you will use these meditations, reflection questions, and prayers to draw closer to Jesus through Mary. Mary leads us to Jesus, just as the blessings of our own child's life can draw us closer to Jesus. Before they can do that, however, we have to recognize and acknowledge them. We have to find those blessings in order to genuinely celebrate, honor, and love our child.

God is perfect love and perfect love drives out fear (see 1 John 4:18). It is scary to look behind the heartache and the struggle of loss and risk finding the blessings. It takes courage to be joyful and to lean on hope. Without fear, however, it is much easier to see the blessings of our child's life.

What fears are you holding on to? Are they keeping you from seeing the blessings of your child's life?

Pray this decade for all who are afraid, that they may be brave enough to open their eyes and see the blessings of God.

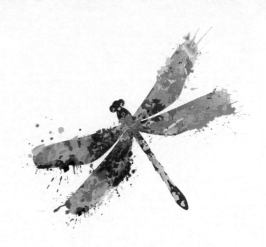

Descent of the Holy Spirit

And suddenly a sound came from heaven like the rush go a mighty wind,
and it filled all the house where they were sitting.

ACTS 2:2

The Holy Spirit was sent from heaven not just for the apostles, but for us! The Holy Spirit is here in our lives, infusing the whole house where we are sitting, mine as I write these words, and yours as you read them.

It is not easy to train ourselves to listen to the voice of the Holy Spirit. He works in many mysterious ways, including through the lives of others. We are interconnected by his workings.

From the moment we learned of Siena's health issues, we prayed specifically to St. Gianna because one of her canonization miracles was related to a baby who survived for many weeks without any amniotic fluid. We asked friends and family to pray for her intercession as well. One day we had a phone call from a friend who had contacted a semi-local Marian shrine with a minor shrine to St. Gianna. The shrine had a pair of St. Gianna's gloves, and they were willing to send a staffer to drive them an hour and a half one way for us to have a time of veneration and prayer as a family. The Holy Spirit made connections through the lives of several individuals to make this happen for us.

Where have you seen the workings of the Holy Spirit on your journey? Think back to previous meditations: who have been your Simons and your Marys? The Holy Spirit has used those people to provide you with comfort, friendship, and physical assistance.

Pray for the surrounding of the Holy Spirit for all who have lost a child.

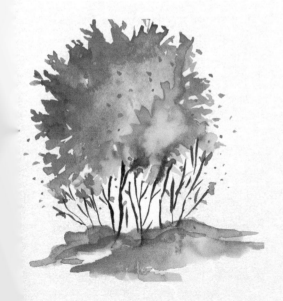

Assumption

The Most Blessed Virgin Mary, when the course of her earthly life
was completed, was taken up body and soul into the glory of heaven,
where she already shares in the glory of her Son's Resurrection,
anticipating the resurrection of all members of his body.

CATECHISM OF THE CATHOLIC CHURCH, #974

Mary was given the grace of achieving the goal of heavenly glory and a share in the resurrection. Don't we all strive for those things? The grace of a happy death. The eternal happiness of heaven. Mary is once again the human model for what we all hope for.

Mary was carried into heaven by her love for Jesus and by his love for her. You might say she was loved into heaven. It is a beautiful and humbling thing to walk with someone on his or her final journey from this earth, to be present in the final days, hours, and even in the final moment.

I have been forever changed by the opportunity to love my daughter Siena into heaven, to see her at peace and to share her with friends and family. Words can't adequately describe what that day was like. My friend Leigh explains, "There is something profound about holding such a tiny body—it made her life, though brief, so very real . . . . Similarly, having extensive pictures . . . has helped remind us all that Siena was and is a person. When my grandpa was dying, it was important for him to hear us say, 'It's okay to let go.' Perhaps it's the reverse for an infant—having the chance to create memories and acknowledge her existence are ways to hold on to the idea that she is real and not let her die, in a sense." *

No matter how long a child lives, it is an incredibly beautiful and important thing to participate with your spouse in the creation of new life. The kind of love that led to the creation of your child can also carry your child and yourself to heaven with the grace f a happy death.

How have you carried your child to heaven with your love? How is he or she carrying you?

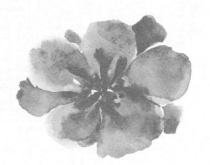

Pray for the grace of a happy death and the goal of eternal happiness.

*You can read more about Leigh's experience with Siena, and also about my friend Lisa's perspective, on the Work and Play Day by Day blog.

Coronation of Mary

And a great sign appeared in heaven, a woman clothed with the sun,
with the moon under her feet, and on her head a crown of twelve stars.

REVELATION 12:1

Upon her assumption into heaven, the Blessed Virgin Mary was crowned as the queen of heaven. There, under her title Mother of the Unborn, she waits to guide and care for our little ones just as she guides and cares for us. As a mother, she too underwent great sorrow in the life of her son. In loving and parenting our Lord, her heart was pierced by a sword.

There are many days, as parents of a child who has died before we could get to know her, that our hearts too are pierced by a sword, days when it does not seem possible to even think or hope for heaven ourselves. In truth, however, it is exactly through the hope of heaven and the comfort of Mary that our own hearts will begin to heal. Our Blessed Mother did not shrink away from the sorrows that awaited her, and great was her heavenly reward.

As we begin to look past our loss experiences and integrate our child's death into our daily lives, it is possible to develop a spiritual relationship with our child. Praying for and seeking the intercession of this child of ours is a meaningful and important thing to do. If you are unsure how to do this, ask our Blessed Mother and she will come to your assistance and help you.

Mary's intercession leads us closer to Jesus and so can your child. Whispers of intercession throughout your day or in particular times of trial can help you feel close to your child and develop this relationship. I sometimes like to remind myself that my girls who died have experienced a much greater understanding of the spiritual mysteries than I can at this time in my life.

How are you developing a spiritual relationship with your child? Ask your child to intercede for you, showing you new ways to draw closer to Christ through your experiences.

Boldly pray this decade of the rosary for full and complete acceptance of your child's life and death and for a fulfilling spiritual relationship with him or her.

When Hope Seems Lost, Hope is Only Beginning

The story of the smallest souls can have the greatest impact. The lives and love of these little ones can draw us closer to Christ in our own walk of faith. It is an undeniably painful process. I do not know one mom who can tell me that her child's death is no longer painful, even if it happened many decades ago.

On the other hand, I know many moms who will also tell me that they have found peace and a new level of spiritual maturity and understanding following their pregnancy or infant loss. Sometimes our life is influenced by our faith and other times our faith is influenced by our life.

Our children's stories may never be known outside of the small circles we are a part of. And yet, through the life that we live our children's legacy continues to live on. We are who we are because of them. Our faith is what it is because of them.

Wherever you are today, my prayer is that you will open yourself to hope. Open your heart to healing and the hope of a future that includes a new spiritual relationship with Mary, Jesus, and also with your child.

There are many in our world who do not want you to share your child. There are some, in fact, who would tell you there is nothing to share and definitely nothing to grieve. That's an unfortunate truth of our society today. I want to encourage you to resist those who would tell you that your child's life does not have value, or that you are weak for loving your little one. Never be afraid to share your child's life with a friend. Mary can be that friend. She loves your child as much as she loves you and is waiting to hear from you.

Immaculate Heart of Mary, pray for us.
Sacred Heart of Jesus, have mercy on us.

Resources

Curley, Terence P. *Six Steps for Managing Loss: A Catholic Guide Through Grief.* Staten Island, NY: Alba House, 1997.

Currie, Colleen and David B. *Loving Baby Louie.* Steubenville, Ohio: Emmaus Road Publishing, 2015.

Flynn, Vinny. *7 Secrets of the Eucharist.* San Francisco: Ignatius Press, 2007.

Kuebelbeck, Amy. *Waiting with Gabriel.* Chicago: Loyola Press, 2008.

Prenatal Partners for Life. *Our Baby Died and Went to Heaven.* (Website listed below.)

Prenatal Partners for Life website: prenatalpartnersforlife.org.

Windley-Daoust, Jerry. *The Illuminated Rosary Series.* Winona, Minn.: PB & Grace, 2015.

https://www.ewtn.com/library/DOCTRINE/BAPTISM.TXT

http://catholicexchange.com/meditations-on-the-rosary-and-miscarriage

"Baby Louie: A Tale of Faith, Hope, & Love."
http://www.catholicsistas.com/2014/10/
baby-louie-a-tale-of-faith-hope-and-love/

"Mallory: God Had Another Plan."
http://www.catholicsistas.com/2013/10/mallory-god-another-plan/

"Miscarriage and Stillbirth: Grieving the Child Who Goes With God."
http://www.pbgrace.com/birth-18/

"Siena's Story: Leigh's Perspective."
http://www.workandplaydaybyday.com/2015/05/sienas-story-leighs-perspective.html

"Siena's Story: Lisa's Perspective."
http://www.workandplaydaybyday.com/2015/10/sienas-story-lisas-perspective.html

"Work and Play, Day by Day: Remembering."
http://www.workandplaydaybyday.com/p/sienastrong.html

[T]he Catechism teaches that infants who die without baptism are entrusted by the Church to the mercy of God, as is shown in the specific funeral rite for such children. The principle that God desires the salvation of all people gives rise to the hope that there is a path to salvation for infants who die without baptism (cf. CCC, 1261), and therefore also to the theological desire to find a coherent and logical connection between the diverse affirmations of the Catholic faith: the universal salvific will of God; the unicity of the mediation of Christ; the necessity of baptism for salvation; the universal action of grace in relation to the sacraments; the link between original sin and the deprivation of the beatific vision; the creation of man "in Christ."

The conclusion of this study is that there are theological and liturgical reasons to hope that infants who die without baptism may be saved and brought into eternal happiness, even if there is not an explicit teaching on this question found in Revelation.

—International Theological Commission,
The Hope of Salvation for Infants Who Die Without Baptism